Bodybuilding diet cookbook for women 2024

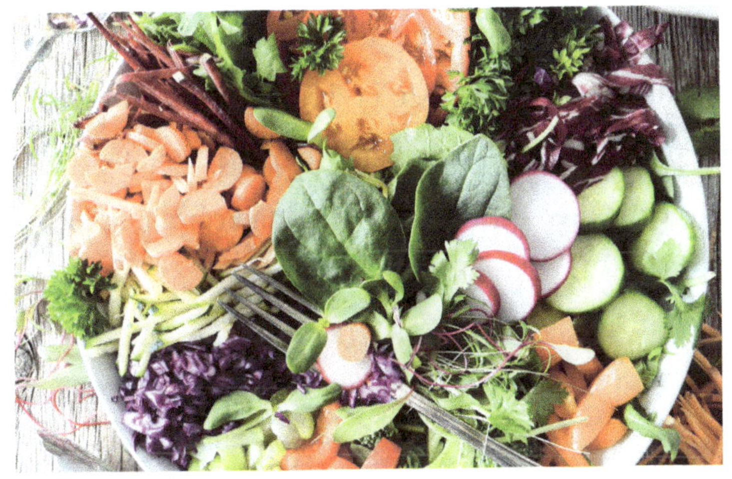

Over +30 Recipes for Building Muscle, Getting Lean, live longer and Staying Healthy

Misty J. Font

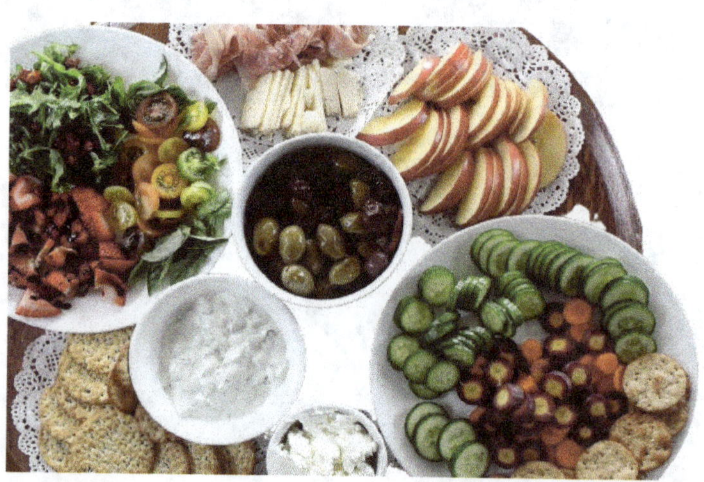

Table of contents

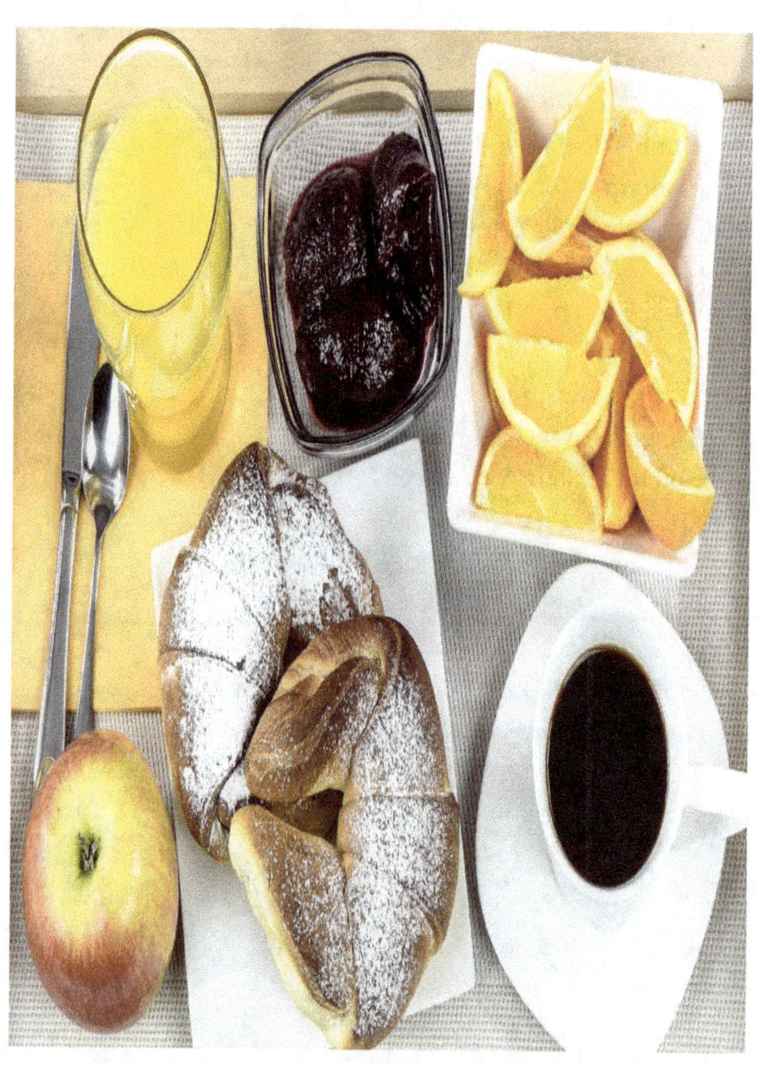

Introduction

In the heart of the city, amidst the whirlwind of deadlines and demands, Jennifer found herself yearning for a change—a change that would not only transform her body but also nourish her soul. For years, she had struggled with her relationship with food, alternating between strict dieting and indulgent bingeing, all while feeling trapped in a cycle of guilt and shame. But deep down, she knew there had to be a better way—a way to provide her body with the nutrients it craved without causing deprivation or restriction.

Enter the bodybuilding diet cookbook for women, a beacon of hope in Jennifer's quest for health and happiness. As she flipped through the pages of vibrant photographs and tantalizing recipes, she felt a surge of excitement rise within her. Nestled among the glossy pages were the tools she needed to reset her relationship with food and embark on a journey of self-discovery.

Jennifer dove headfirst into the world of bodybuilding nutrition, eager to learn the secrets of optimal health and vitality, guided by the cookbook. The days of counting calories and obsessing over portion sizes were over; instead, she learned to see food as fuel for her body, providing it with the nutrients it required to thrive.

Each recipe in the cookbook was a culinary masterpiece, meticulously crafted to achieve the ideal ratio of protein, carbohydrates, and fats. Every dish, from hearty breakfast bowls bursting with fresh fruits and grains to savory stir-fries packed with lean proteins and vibrant vegetables, demonstrated the power of wholesome, nutrient-dense ingredients.

However, the cookbook was more than just a collection of recipes; it also served as a road map for Jennifer's journey of self-discovery. With each meal she prepared, she found herself reconnecting with her body and acknowledging its enormous potential. The days of mindless eating and emotional binging were over; instead, she savored each bite mindfully, relishing the flavors and textures that danced across her palette.

As Jennifer worked her way through the cookbook, she felt a surge of empowerment and confidence. She no longer felt constrained by restrictive dieting and adopted a more flexible approach to nutrition, allowing herself to indulge in her favorite treats without guilt or shame. And with each passing day, she felt herself becoming stronger, both physically and mentally, as she fed her body with love and respect.

Perhaps the most profound transformation occurred within Jennifer's soul. As she adopted bodybuilding nutrition principles, she found herself losing not only weight but also layers of self-doubt and insecurity. In their place, she discovered a renewed sense of self-worth and acceptance as she learned to love herself unconditionally, flaws and all.

Understanding Body building Nutrition

Tools and Techniques for Success

Arming yourself with the proper tools and techniques is essential for success in any endeavor, including bodybuilding. In this section, we will look at a variety of strategies to help you stay on track and achieve your goals. From meal planning and prepping to incorporating supplements and superfoods into your diet, you'll learn practical tips and tricks for improving your nutrition and achieving your goals. With the right tools and techniques at your disposal, you'll be well-prepared to overcome any obstacles in your path and emerge stronger than ever.

As you embark on this journey with "Strong & Sculpted," I encourage you to be open-minded and willing to embrace change. Remember that transformation is more than just changing your body; it also entails changing your mindset, habits, and lifestyle in order to become the best version of yourself. So, let's dive in together and unleash your inner strength and power. Your journey to a stronger, more sculpted you begins now.

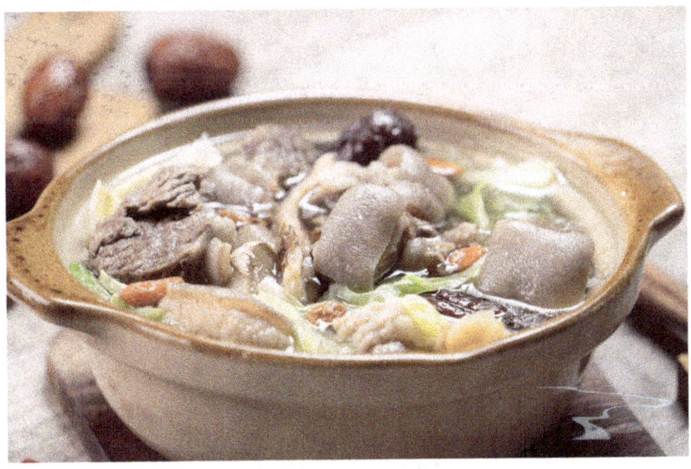

Chapter 1: Fueling Your Workouts

Welcome to Chapter 1 of "Strong & Sculpted: The Ultimate Bodybuilding Cookbook for Women," where we will cover the critical topic of fueling your workouts for maximum performance and results. Whether you're hitting the gym for an intense weightlifting session or powering through a high-intensity interval training (HIIT) workout, what you eat before, during, and after exercise has a significant impact on your ability to perform well and recover efficiently.

Pre-Workout Nutrition Essentials

Your pre-workout meal sets the tone for success by providing your body with the energy it requires to power through your workout. In this section, we'll look at the key components of a pre-workout meal, such as the importance of carbohydrates for energy, the role of protein in muscle repair and growth, and the importance of timing your meals for peak performance. From quick and easy snacks to more substantial meals, you'll find a wide range of pre-workout nutrition options to suit your preferences and dietary requirements.

Post-Workout Recovery Meals

Once you've completed your workout, it's time to focus on recovery and replenishment. Post-workout nutrition is critical for muscle repair, glycogen replenishment, and overall recovery. In this section, we'll go over how important it is to consume a combination of protein and carbohydrates during the post-workout window in order to improve recovery and muscle growth. You'll find a variety of delicious and nutritious post-workout meal options designed to refuel your body and help you recover faster, allowing you to return to training feeling stronger than ever.

Proper hydration is commonly overlooked, but it is critical for peak performance and overall health. Dehydration can cause low energy levels, impaired cognitive function, and decreased exercise performance. In this section, we'll look at how important it is to stay hydrated before, during, and after your workouts, as well as practical tips for meeting your fluid needs. From calculating your hydration needs to incorporating hydrating foods and beverages into your diet, you'll learn how to prioritize hydration to help you reach your fitness goals and perform at your best.

As you read Chapter 1 of "Strong & Sculpted," keep in mind that nutrition is the cornerstone of your fitness success. By fueling your workouts with the right nutrients and staying hydrated, you'll set yourself up for success and maximize your growth and progress potential. So let's fuel up, crush those workouts, and get one step closer to having the strong, sculpted physique you've always desired.

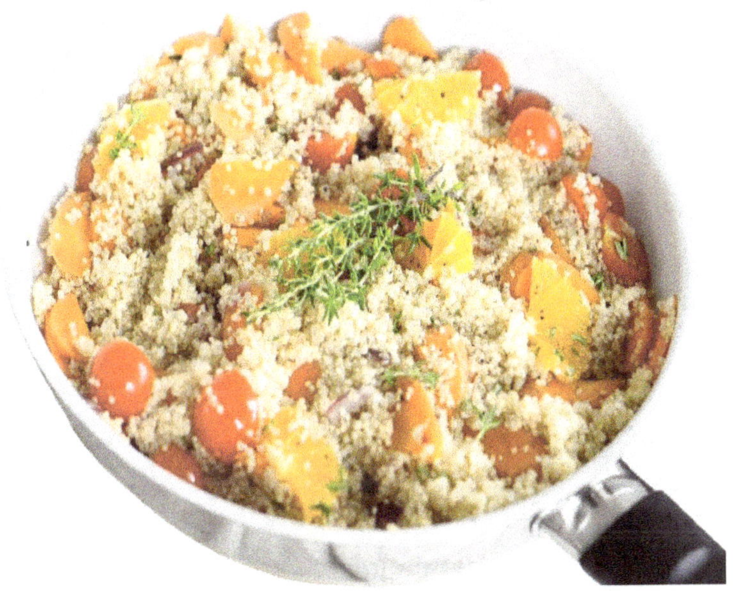

Chapter 2: Protein-packed Breakfasts

Egg White Veggie Scramble

This delicious egg white veggie scramble will give you a protein and nutrient boost to start the day. It's a filling and healthy breakfast option that includes colorful vegetables and lean protein.

Serving Size: 1
Prep Time: 5 minutes
Cooking Time: 10 minutes

Ingredients:

- 1 cup egg whites
- 1/2 cup diced bell peppers (any color)
- 1/4 cup diced onions
- 1/4 cup chopped spinach
- Salt and pepper to taste

- Cooking spray or olive oil for the pan

Instructions:

1. Heat a nonstick skillet over medium heat and coat with cooking spray or a small amount of olive oil.
2. Sauté the diced bell peppers and onions in the skillet for about 3-4 minutes, or until softened.
3. Cook the chopped spinach in the skillet until wilted, which should take about 1-2 minutes.
4. Add the egg whites and season with salt and pepper.
5. Cook, stirring occasionally, until the eggs are fully cooked and scrambled, about 3-4 minutes.
6. Serve hot, and enjoy!

Greek Yogurt Parfait

This protein-rich Greek yogurt parfait is a tasty and nutritious way to begin the day. Layered with creamy yogurt, fresh fruit, and crunchy granola, this breakfast will keep you full and energized.

Serving Size: 1
Prep Time: 5 minutes

Ingredients:

- 1/2 cup plain Greek yogurt
- 1/4 cup fresh berries (such as strawberries, blueberries, or raspberries)
- 1/4 cup granola
- 1 tablespoon honey or maple syrup (optional)

Instructions:

1. In a serving glass or bowl, place half of the Greek yogurt.

2. Place half of the fresh berries on top of the yogurt.

3. Sprinkle half of the granola over the berries.

4. Repeat the layers with the remaining yogurt, berries, and granola.

5. Drizzle with honey or maple syrup as desired.

6. Serve immediately and enjoy!

Spinach and Feta Egg Muffins

These spinach and feta egg muffins make an excellent meal prep option or a quick breakfast on the go. They're a delicious and nutritious way to start the day, with plenty of protein and vegetables.

Serving Size: 2 muffins

Prep Time: 10 minutes

Cooking Time: 20 minutes

Ingredients:

- 6 large eggs

- 1 cup chopped spinach

- 1/4 cup crumbled feta cheese

- Salt and pepper to taste

- Cooking spray or olive oil for the muffin tin

Instructions:

1. Preheat the oven to 350°F/175°C and lightly grease a muffin tin with cooking spray or olive oil.

2. In a mixing bowl, whisk the eggs until well combined.

3. Stir in the chopped spinach and crumbled feta cheese until well combined.

4. Season with salt and pepper to taste.

5. Pour the egg mixture into the muffin cups, filling them about 3/4 full.

6. Bake in the preheated oven for 18-20 minutes, or until the egg muffins are firm and lightly golden on top.

7. Remove from the oven and let cool for a few minutes before serving.

8. Serve warm or refrigerate in an airtight container for up to three days. Enjoy!

Protein-Packed Breakfast Burrito

This protein-packed breakfast burrito is the ideal way to prepare for the day ahead. It's a filling and nutritious meal that takes only a few minutes to prepare.

Serving Size: 1
Prep Time: 10 minutes
Cooking Time: 10 minutes

Ingredients:
- 2 large eggs
- 1/4 cup black beans, drained and rinsed
- 1/4 avocado, sliced
- 2 tablespoons shredded cheddar cheese

- 1 small whole wheat or corn tortilla
- Salt and pepper to taste
- Salsa, for serving (optional)

Instructions:

1. In a small bowl, beat the eggs until well combined. Season with salt and pepper to taste.

2. Heat a nonstick skillet over medium heat and coat with cooking spray or a small amount of olive oil.

3. Pour the beaten eggs into the skillet and cook, stirring occasionally, until scrambled and thoroughly cooked, about 3-4 minutes.

4. Heat the tortilla in a skillet or microwave for a few seconds until pliable.

5. Place the scrambled eggs in the middle of the tortilla.

6. Add black beans, avocado slices, and shredded cheddar cheese.

7. Fold the tortilla's sides over the filling and roll it up like a burrito.

8. Serve immediately, with salsa on the side if you like. Enjoy!

Quinoa Breakfast Bowl

This quinoa breakfast bowl is a satisfying and nutritious way to begin the day. It's a delicious and satisfying meal that is high in protein, fiber, and essential nutrients, keeping you full and energized until lunchtime.

Serving Size: 1
Prep Time: 5 minutes
Cooking Time: 15 minutes

Ingredients:

- 1/2 cup cooked quinoa
- 1/4 cup sliced almonds
- 1/4 cup Greek yogurt

- 1/4 cup fresh berries (such as strawberries, blueberries, or raspberries)
- 1 tablespoon honey or maple syrup (optional)

Instructions:

1. In a small saucepan, warm the cooked quinoa over medium heat for about 2-3 minutes.
2. Transfer the warm quinoa to a serving bowl.
3. Garnish with sliced almonds, Greek yogurt, and fresh berries.
4. Drizzle with honey or maple syrup as desired.
5. Serve immediately and enjoy!

Banana Protein Smoothie

This creamy banana protein smoothie is a quick and tasty way to fuel your morning. It's a filling and nutritious breakfast option, thanks to the protein in the Greek yogurt and almond butter.

Serving Size: 1

Prep Time: 5 minutes

Ingredients:

- 1 ripe banana, peeled and sliced
- 1/2 cup plain Greek yogurt
- 1 tablespoon almond butter
- 1/2 cup almond milk (or any milk of your choice)
- 1 scoop protein powder (vanilla or unflavored)
- Ice cubes (optional)

Instructions:

1. Put all of the ingredients in a blender.
2. Blend until smooth and creamy.
3. If desired, add ice cubes to make the smoothie colder.
4. Pour into a glass and drink immediately!

Protein-Packed Breakfast Wrap

This protein-rich breakfast wrap is ideal for a busy morning on the go. Scrambled eggs, turkey bacon, avocado, and cheese make for a filling and portable meal that will keep you going until lunchtime.

Serving Size: 1
Prep Time: 10 minutes
Cooking Time: 5 minutes

Ingredients:
- 2 large eggs, scrambled
- 2 slices turkey bacon, cooked
- 1/4 avocado, sliced
- 1/4 cup shredded cheddar cheese
- 1 small whole wheat or spinach tortilla
- Salt and pepper to taste

Instructions:

1. Heat the tortilla in a skillet or microwave for a few seconds until it is pliable.

2. Place the scrambled eggs in the middle of the tortilla.

3. Garnish with cooked turkey bacon, avocado slices, and shredded cheddar cheese.

4. Season with salt and pepper to taste.

5. Fold the tortilla's sides over the filling, then roll it up into a wrap.

6. Serve immediately or wrap in foil for a convenient breakfast option.

Protein-Packed Oatmeal

This protein-rich oatmeal is a comforting and nutritious breakfast choice that will keep you full and satisfied all morning. It's simple to make and delicious to eat, consisting of rolled oats, protein powder, and your favorite toppings.

Serving Size: 1

Prep Time: 5 minutes

Cooking Time: 5 minutes

Ingredients:

- 1/2 cup rolled oats
- 1 cup water or milk (dairy or plant-based)
- 1 scoop protein powder (vanilla or chocolate)
- Toppings of your choice (such as sliced bananas, berries, nuts, seeds, or nut butter)

Instructions:

1. In a small saucepan, heat the water or milk until it boils.
2. Stir in the rolled oats, then reduce the heat to medium-low.
3. Cook, stirring occasionally, for about 3-5 minutes, or until the oats are thick and creamy.
4. Remove from the heat and stir in the protein powder until thoroughly combined.

5. Transfer the oatmeal to a bowl and top with your desired toppings.

6. Serve immediately and enjoy!

High-Protein Breakfast Cookies

These high-protein breakfast cookies are a tasty and convenient way to begin the day. They're a portable breakfast option ideal for busy mornings, made with oats, almond butter, protein powder, and chocolate chips.

Serving Size: 2 cookies

Prep Time: 10 minutes

Cooking Time: 12 minutes

Ingredients:

- 1 cup rolled oats
- 1/2 cup almond butter
- 1/4 cup honey or maple syrup
- 1 scoop protein powder (vanilla or chocolate)

- 1/4 cup dark chocolate chips

Instructions:

1. Preheat the oven to 350°F/175°C and line a baking sheet with parchment paper.

2. In a mixing bowl, mix together the rolled oats, almond butter, honey or maple syrup, protein powder, and chocolate chips. Stir until thoroughly combined.

3. Drop spoonfuls of cookie dough onto the prepared baking sheet with a cookie scoop or spoon.

4. Flatten each cookie slightly with a spoon or your fingers.

5. Bake the cookies in the preheated oven for 10-12 minutes, or until golden brown on the edges.

6. Remove from the oven and cool for a few minutes on the baking sheet before transferring to a wire rack to finish cooling.

7. After cooling, store the cookies in an airtight
   container at room temperature for up to a
   week.

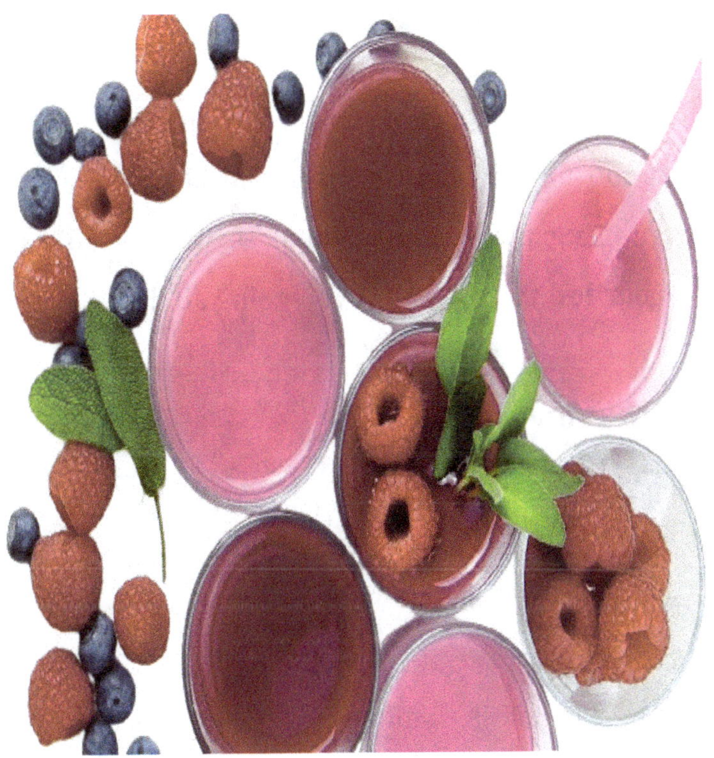

Chapter 3 : High-Protein Lunches for Energy

Grilled Chicken Quinoa Salad

This grilled chicken quinoa salad makes a hearty and nutritious lunch. It's a filling meal full of protein from the chicken and quinoa, as well as colorful vegetables, that will keep you going all day.

Serving Size: 2
Prep Time: 15 minutes
Cooking Time: 20 minutes

Ingredients:

- 2 boneless, skinless chicken breasts
- 1 cup quinoa, cooked
- 2 cups mixed greens
- 1 cup cherry tomatoes, halved
- 1 cucumber, diced

- 1/4 red onion, thinly sliced
- 1/4 cup feta cheese, crumbled
- 2 tablespoons olive oil
- 2 tablespoons balsamic vinegar
- Salt and pepper to taste

Instructions:

1. Preheat the grill to medium-high heat.
2. Season chicken breasts with salt and pepper, then grill for 6-8 minutes per side until fully cooked. Rest for a few minutes before slicing.
3. In a large mixing bowl, combine the cooked quinoa, mixed greens, cherry tomatoes, cucumber, red onion, and feta cheese.
4. Make the dressing by whisking olive oil and balsamic vinegar together in a small bowl.
5. Toss the salad with the sliced chicken and the dressing.
6. Divide the salad between two plates and serve immediately.

Turkey and Avocado Wrap

This turkey and avocado wrap is a quick and easy lunch filled with protein and healthy fats. Ideal for a busy day when you require a nutritious meal on the go.

Serving Size: 1
Prep Time: 10 minutes

Ingredients:

- 1 whole wheat or spinach tortilla
- 3 slices turkey breast
- 1/4 avocado, sliced
- 1/4 cup shredded lettuce
- 2 slices tomato
- 1 tablespoon hummus
- Salt and pepper to taste

Instructions:

1. Lay the tortilla flat on a clean surface.

2. Spread the hummus evenly on the tortilla.

3. Place turkey slices, avocado slices, shredded lettuce, and tomato slices on top of the hummus.

4. Season with salt and pepper to taste.

5. Roll the tortilla tightly, then cut in half.

6. Serve immediately or store in foil for later.

Tuna Salad Stuffed Bell Peppers

Tuna salad stuffed bell peppers are a light but protein-rich lunch option. They're both nutritious and tasty, thanks to a flavorful tuna salad filling stuffed into colorful bell peppers.

Serving Size: 2

Prep Time: 15 minutes

Ingredients:

- 2 large bell peppers, halved and seeds removed
- 1 can tuna, drained
- 1/4 cup Greek yogurt
- 1 tablespoon Dijon mustard
- 1/4 cup diced celery
- 1/4 cup diced red onion
- 1 tablespoon chopped fresh dill
- Salt and pepper to taste

Instructions:

1. In a mixing bowl, combine the drained tuna, Greek yogurt, Dijon mustard, diced celery, red onion, and fresh dill.
2. Season to taste with salt and pepper, then mix thoroughly.
3. Spoon the tuna salad mixture evenly into each of the halved bell peppers.
4. Serve immediately or refrigerate until ready to eat.

Quinoa and Black Bean Buddha Bowl

This quinoa and black bean Buddha bowl is a colorful and nutritionally dense lunch option. It's a filling meal with plenty of protein, fiber, and healthy fats to keep you going.

Serving Size: 2
Prep Time: 20 minutes
Cooking Time: 15 minutes

Ingredients:

- 1 cup quinoa, cooked
- 1 can black beans, drained and rinsed
- 1 cup cooked sweet potatoes, diced
- 1 cup cherry tomatoes, halved
- 1/2 cup corn kernels
- 1/4 cup diced red onion
- 1 avocado, sliced
- 1/4 cup cilantro, chopped

- 2 tablespoons lime juice
- 2 tablespoons olive oil
- Salt and pepper to taste

Instructions:

1. In a large mixing bowl, combine cooked quinoa, black beans, diced sweet potatoes, cherry tomatoes, corn kernels, and diced red onion.
2. Make the dressing by whisking together lime juice, olive oil, salt, and pepper in a small bowl.
3. Drizzle dressing over quinoa and black bean mixture, then toss to combine.
4. Divide the quinoa mixture into two bowls.
5. Top each bowl with sliced avocado and cilantro.
6. Serve immediately or refrigerate until ready to eat.

Grilled Salmon Salad

This grilled salmon salad is a light and refreshing lunch option rich in protein and omega-3 fatty acids. Ideal for a warm day when you want something nutritious and filling.

Serving Size: 2
Prep Time: 10 minutes
Cooking Time: 10 minutes

Ingredients:

- 2 salmon fillets
- 4 cups mixed greens
- 1 cup cherry tomatoes, halved
- 1/2 cucumber, sliced
- 1/4 red onion, thinly sliced
- 1/4 cup sliced almonds
- 2 tablespoons olive oil
- 2 tablespoons lemon juice

- Salt and pepper to taste

Instructions:

1. Preheat the grill to medium-high heat.
2. Season the salmon fillets with salt, pepper, and a drizzle of olive oil.
3. Grill salmon fillets for 4-5 minutes on each side, or until cooked through and flaky.
4. In a large mixing bowl, combine mixed greens, cherry tomatoes, cucumber, thinly sliced red onion, and sliced almonds.
5. To prepare the dressing, combine olive oil, lemon juice, salt, and pepper in a small bowl.
6. Drizzle dressing over salad and toss to coat.
7. Divide the salad between two plates, and top each with a grilled salmon fillet.
8. Serve immediately and enjoy!

Mediterranean Chickpea Salad

This Mediterranean chickpea salad is a delicious and protein-rich lunch option. With chickpeas, vegetables, and feta cheese tossed in a tangy vinaigrette, it's a filling meal for any day of the week.

Serving Size: 2
Prep Time: 15 minutes

Ingredients:

- 1 can chickpeas, drained and rinsed
- 1 cup cucumber, diced
- 1 cup cherry tomatoes, halved
- 1/4 cup red onion, thinly sliced
- 1/4 cup Kalamata olives, sliced
- 1/4 cup crumbled feta cheese
- 2 tablespoons fresh parsley, chopped
- 2 tablespoons olive oil

- 1 tablespoon red wine vinegar
- 1 teaspoon dried oregano
- Salt and pepper to taste

Instructions:

1. In a large mixing bowl, combine the chickpeas, diced cucumber, halved cherry tomatoes, thinly sliced red onion, sliced Kalamata olives, crumbled feta cheese, and chopped fresh parsley.
2. To prepare the dressing, combine olive oil, red wine vinegar, dried oregano, salt, and pepper in a small bowl.
3. Toss the salad mixture with the dressing until coated.
4. Divide the salad between two plates and serve immediately.

Soy Ginger Tofu Stir-Fry

This soy ginger tofu stir-fry is a flavorful and protein-packed lunch option that comes together in minutes. It's a filling meal with crispy tofu, colorful vegetables, and a tangy ginger sauce that's ideal for busy days.

Serving Size: 2
Prep Time: 15 minutes
Cooking Time: 15 minutes

Ingredients:

- 1 block extra firm tofu, pressed and cubed
- 2 tablespoons soy sauce
- 1 tablespoon sesame oil
- 1 tablespoon cornstarch
- 2 cloves garlic, minced
- 1 tablespoon fresh ginger, grated

- 2 cups mixed vegetables (such as bell peppers, broccoli, carrots, and snap peas)
- Cooked brown rice or quinoa, for serving

Instructions:

1. In a small bowl, combine soy sauce, sesame oil, and cornstarch to make the sauce.

2. Heat a large skillet or wok over medium heat. Add the cubed tofu. Cook for approximately 8-10 minutes, or until crispy and golden brown on all sides. Remove the tofu from the skillet and set aside.

3. In the same skillet, combine the minced garlic and grated ginger. Cook for one to two minutes, or until fragrant.

4. Stir-fry the mixed vegetables in the skillet for about 5-7 minutes, or until they are tender and crisp.

5. Return the cooked tofu to the skillet and pour the sauce over the vegetables. Stir thoroughly to coat.

6. Cook for an additional 2-3 minutes, or until the sauce thickens and everything is thoroughly heated.

7. Serve stir-fry with cooked brown rice or quinoa.

Turkey and Quinoa Stuffed Bell Peppers

Turkey and quinoa stuffed bell peppers are a protein-rich and nutritious lunch option. They're a delicious and filling meal that's ideal for meal prep, with lean ground turkey, quinoa, vegetables, and melted cheese on top.

Serving Size: 2

Prep Time: 20 minutes

Cooking Time: 40 minutes

Ingredients:

- 4 large bell peppers, halved and seeds removed
- 1/2 cup quinoa, cooked
- 1/2 pound lean ground turkey
- 1/2 cup onion, diced
- 1/2 cup bell pepper, diced
- 1 clove garlic, minced
- 1 teaspoon Italian seasoning
- Salt and pepper to taste
- 1/2 cup tomato sauce
- 1/2 cup shredded mozzarella cheese

Instructions:

1. Preheat the oven to 375° Fahrenheit (190° Celsius).
2. Cook ground turkey in a large skillet over medium heat until browned and fully cooked. If necessary, drain off any excess fat.

3. Add diced onion, diced bell pepper, minced garlic, Italian seasoning, salt, and pepper to the skillet. Cook for approximately 5-7 minutes, or until the vegetables have softened.

4. Stir in the cooked quinoa and tomato sauce until thoroughly combined.

5. Place the halved bell peppers in a baking dish, cut side up.

6. Spoon the turkey and quinoa mixture into each bell pepper half.

7. Bake in a preheated oven for 30 minutes.

8. Remove the foil, then top the stuffed peppers with shredded mozzarella cheese and bake for another 5-10 minutes, or until melted and bubbly.

9. Serve the stuffed bell peppers hot.

Shrimp and Avocado Salad

This shrimp and avocado salad is a light and refreshing lunch filled with protein and healthy fats. With juicy shrimp, creamy avocado, and crisp vegetables, it's a filling meal ideal for warmer weather.

Serving Size: 2
Prep Time: 15 minutes
Cooking Time: 5 minutes

Ingredients:

- 1 pound shrimp, peeled and deveined
- 1 tablespoon olive oil
- 1 teaspoon chili powder
- Salt and pepper to taste
- 4 cups mixed greens
- 1 avocado, diced
- 1/2 cup cherry tomatoes, halved

- 1/4 cup red onion, thinly sliced
- 1/4 cup cilantro, chopped
- 2 tablespoons lime juice
- 1 tablespoon olive oil

Instructions:

1. In a large skillet, heat the olive oil over medium heat.
2. Season the shrimp with chili powder, salt, and pepper, then place in the skillet.
3. Cook shrimp for 2-3 minutes on each side, or until pink and opaque.
4. In a large mixing bowl, combine mixed greens, diced avocado, halved cherry tomatoes, thinly sliced red onion, and chopped cilantro.
5. To prepare the dressing, whisk together lime juice and olive oil in a small bowl.
6. Toss cooked shrimp into the salad mixture, then drizzle with dressing to coat.

7. Divide the salad between two plates and serve immediately.

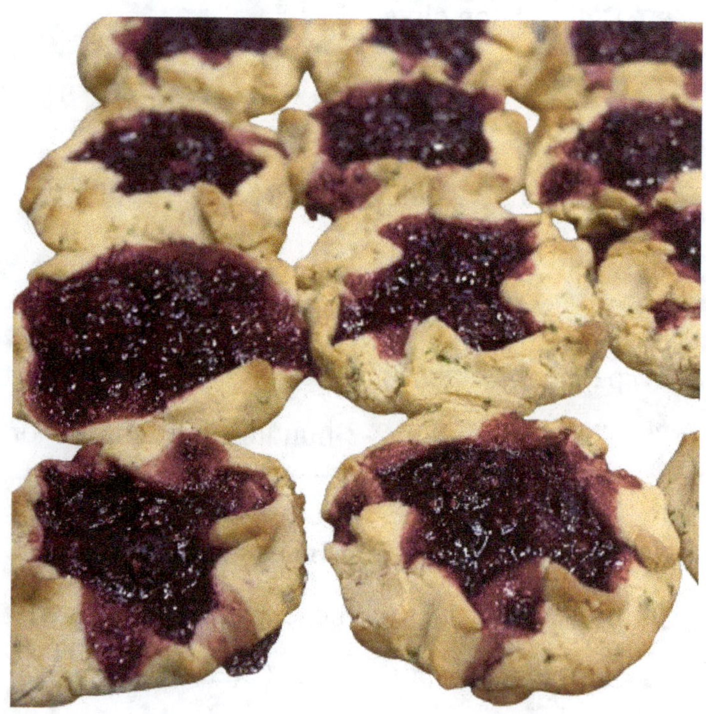

Chapter 4: Muscle-Building Dinners to Refuel

Grilled Steak with Sweet Potato Mash

This grilled steak with sweet potato mash is a hearty and filling dinner that's ideal for fueling up after a strenuous workout. With tender grilled steak and creamy sweet potato mash, it's high in protein and complex carbohydrates to help you refuel.

Serving Size: 2
Prep Time: 15 minutes
Cooking Time: 20 minutes

Ingredients:

- 2 sirloin steaks
- 2 large sweet potatoes, peeled and diced
- 2 tablespoons olive oil
- Salt and pepper to taste

- 2 tablespoons butter (optional)
- 1/4 cup milk (optional)

Instructions:

1. Preheat the grill to medium-high heat.
2. Rub olive oil on the steaks and season with salt and pepper.
3. Grill the steaks for 4-5 minutes on each side, or until done to your liking.
4. Meanwhile, cook sweet potatoes in a pot of water until fork tender, about 10-15 minutes.
5. Drain the sweet potatoes and mash with a potato masher or fork.
6. If desired, add butter and milk to make the mash creamier.
7. Serve grilled steaks with sweet potato mash on the side.

Baked Lemon Herb Salmon with Quinoa

This baked lemon herb salmon with quinoa is a light but filling dinner full of protein and healthy fats. With flaky salmon fillets and fluffy quinoa, this nutritious meal is ideal for refueling after a workout.

Serving Size: 2
Prep Time: 10 minutes
Cooking Time: 20 minutes

Ingredients:

- 2 salmon fillets
- 1 lemon, sliced
- 2 tablespoons olive oil
- 2 cloves garlic, minced
- à1 teaspoon dried thyme
- 1 teaspoon dried rosemary
- Salt and pepper to taste
- 1 cup quinoa, cooked

- Fresh parsley for garnish

Instructions:

1. Preheat the oven to 375° Fahrenheit (190° Celsius).

2. Place the salmon fillets on a parchment-lined baking sheet.

3. Drizzle olive oil over salmon fillets, then sprinkle with minced garlic, dried thyme, dried rosemary, salt, and pepper.

4. Place lemon slices on top of each salmon fillet.

5. Bake salmon in a preheated oven for 15-20 minutes, or until cooked through and easily flaked with a fork.

6. Meanwhile, cook the quinoa according to the package instructions.

7. Serve the baked salmon with cooked quinoa on the side.

8. Garnish with fresh parsley before serving.

Grilled Chicken Breast with Roasted Vegetables

This grilled chicken breast with roasted vegetables is a simple and nutritious dinner option that's ideal for replenishing energy after a workout. With juicy grilled chicken and a variety of colorful vegetables, this is a well-balanced meal high in protein and essential nutrients.

Serving Size: 2
Prep Time: 15 minutes
Cooking Time: 25 minutes

Ingredients:
- 2 boneless, skinless chicken breasts
- 2 cups mixed vegetables (such as bell peppers, zucchini, carrots, and red onion), chopped
- 2 tablespoons olive oil

- 1 teaspoon garlic powder
- 1 teaspoon dried oregano
- Salt and pepper to taste

Instructions:

1. Preheat the grill to medium-high heat.
2. Rub olive oil over chicken breasts and season with garlic powder, dried oregano, salt, and pepper.
3. Grill chicken breasts for 6-8 minutes per side, or until thoroughly cooked and no longer pink in the center.
4. Meanwhile, preheat the oven to 400°F (200° C).
5. On a parchment-lined baking sheet, toss the vegetables with olive oil, salt, and pepper.
6. Roast vegetables in a preheated oven for 15-20 minutes, or until they are tender and lightly browned.

7. Serve grilled chicken breasts with roasted vegetables on the side.

Beef and Broccoli Stir-Fry

This beef and broccoli stir-fry is a quick and nutritious dinner filled with protein and vegetables. Tender beef slices, crisp broccoli florets, and a savory sauce make for a delicious post-workout meal.

Serving Size: 2
Prep Time: 15 minutes
Cooking Time: 15 minutes

Ingredients:

- 1/2 pound flank steak, thinly sliced
- 2 cups broccoli florets
- 1 tablespoon olive oil
- 2 cloves garlic, minced
- 1 teaspoon fresh ginger, grated

- 1/4 cup low-sodium soy sauce
- 2 tablespoons hoisin sauce
- 1 tablespoon cornstarch
- Cooked brown rice, for serving

Instructions:

1. To prepare the sauce, combine soy sauce, hoisin sauce, and cornstarch in a small bowl. Set aside.
2. Heat the olive oil in a large skillet or wok over medium-high heat.
3. Cook the sliced flank steak in the skillet until browned, about 2-3 minutes per side. Remove the steak from the skillet and set aside.
4. In the same skillet, combine the minced garlic and grated ginger. Cook for one to two minutes, or until fragrant.
5. Cook the broccoli florets in the skillet for 3-4 minutes, or until they are tender and crisp.

6. Return the cooked steak to the skillet and pour the sauce over the beef and broccoli mixture. Stir thoroughly to coat.

7. Cook for an additional 2-3 minutes, or until the sauce thickens and everything is thoroughly heated.

8. Serve the beef and broccoli stir-fry with cooked brown rice.

Baked Chicken Parmesan

This baked chicken Parmesan is a healthier alternative to the traditional Italian dish. Crispy baked chicken breasts topped with marinara sauce and melted mozzarella cheese make for a delicious and protein-packed dinner that's ideal for refueling after a workout.

Serving Size: 2

Prep Time: 15 minutes

Cooking Time: 25 minutes

Ingredients:

- 2 boneless, skinless chicken breasts
- 1/2 cup breadcrumbs
- 1/4 cup grated Parmesan cheese
- 1 teaspoon Italian seasoning
- 1/2 cup marinara sauce
- 1/2 cup shredded mozzarella cheese
- Fresh basil for garnish

Instructions:

1. Preheat the oven to 400° F (200° C).
2. In a shallow dish, mix together breadcrumbs, grated Parmesan cheese, and Italian seasoning.
3. Dip each chicken breast into the breadcrumb mixture and press to coat evenly.
4. Place the breaded chicken breasts on a parchment-lined baking sheet.

5. Bake chicken breasts in a preheated oven for 20 minutes.

6. Remove the chicken breasts from the oven and spread marinara sauce over each.

7. Add shredded mozzarella cheese to the marinara sauce.

8. Return the chicken breasts to the oven and cook for another 5 minutes, or until the cheese is melted and bubbling.

9. Garnish with fresh basil before serving.

Tofu and Vegetable Stir-Fry

This tofu and vegetable stir-fry is a flavorful and nutrient-dense dinner option. It's a filling meal with crispy tofu cubes, colorful vegetables, and a savory sauce, ideal for refueling after a workout.

Serving Size: 2

Prep Time: 15 minutes

Cooking Time: 15 minutes

Ingredients:

- 1 block extra firm tofu, pressed and cubed
- 2 tablespoons soy sauce
- 1 tablespoon hoisin sauce
- 1 tablespoon rice vinegar
- 1 teaspoon sesame oil
- 1 tablespoon cornstarch
- 2 tablespoons olive oil
- 2 cloves garlic, minced
- 1 teaspoon fresh ginger, grated
- 2 cups mixed vegetables (such as bell peppers, snap peas, carrots, and broccoli)

Instructions:

1. To prepare the sauce, combine soy sauce, hoisin sauce, rice vinegar, sesame oil, and cornstarch in a small bowl. Set aside.

2. Heat the olive oil in a large skillet or wok over medium-high heat.

3. Cook cubed tofu in the skillet until golden brown and crispy on all sides, about 5-7 minutes. Remove the tofu from the skillet and set aside.

4. In the same skillet, combine the minced garlic and grated ginger. Cook for one to two minutes, or until fragrant.

5. Stir-fry the mixed vegetables in the skillet for 3-4 minutes, or until they are tender and crisp.

6. Return the cooked tofu to the skillet, and then pour the sauce over the vegetables. Stir thoroughly to coat.

7. Cook for an additional 2-3 minutes, or until the sauce thickens and everything is thoroughly heated.

8. Serve the tofu and vegetable stir-fry hot with cooked rice or quinoa.

Salmon and Asparagus Foil Packets

These salmon and asparagus foil packets are a simple yet flavorful dinner option that's perfect for busy weeknights. With tender salmon fillets, crisp asparagus spears, and a tangy lemon herb sauce, it's a nutritious meal that's perfect for refueling after a workout.

Serving Size: 2
Prep Time: 10 minutes
Cooking Time: 20 minutes

Ingredients:

- 2 salmon fillets
- 1 bunch asparagus, trimmed
- 2 tablespoons olive oil
- 1 lemon, sliced
- 2 cloves garlic, minced
- 1 teaspoon dried dill

- Salt and pepper to taste

Instructions:

1. Preheat the oven to 375° Fahrenheit (190° Celsius).

2. Arrange each salmon fillet on a large piece of aluminum foil.

3. Arrange asparagus spears around the salmon fillets.

4. Drizzle the salmon and asparagus with olive oil, then top with minced garlic, dried dill, salt, and pepper.

5. Put lemon slices on top of each salmon fillet.

6. Fold up the edges of the foil to form a packet and seal tightly.

7. Place the foil packets on a baking sheet and bake in the preheated oven for 15-20 minutes, or until the salmon is cooked through and easily flaked with a fork.

8. Carefully open the foil packets to serve the salmon and asparagus hot.

Eggplant and Chickpea Curry

This eggplant and chickpea curry is a flavorful and protein-packed dinner option that's ideal for fueling up after a workout. Tender eggplant, creamy chickpeas, and aromatic spices make for a comforting and satisfying meal that goes well with rice or naan.

Serving Size: 4
Prep Time: 15 minutes
Cooking Time: 30 minutes

Ingredients:

- 1 large eggplant, diced
- 1 can chickpeas, drained and rinsed
- 1 onion, diced
- 2 cloves garlic, minced

- 1 tablespoon ginger, grated
- 1 can diced tomatoes
- 1 can coconut milk
- 2 tablespoons curry powder
- 1 teaspoon ground cumin
- 1 teaspoon ground coriander
- Salt and pepper to taste
- Fresh cilantro for garnish

Instructions:

1. In a large pot or skillet, warm the olive oil over medium heat.

2. Add the diced onion, minced garlic, and grated ginger to the pot. Cook until the onion is translucent, which should take about 3-4 minutes.

3. Combine curry powder, ground cumin, and ground coriander. Cook for another 1-2 minutes, until fragrant.

4. Cook the diced eggplant for 5-7 minutes, or until softened.

5. Stir in the diced tomatoes, chickpeas, and coconut milk. Season with salt and pepper to taste.

6. Simmer the curry for 15-20 minutes, or until the eggplant is tender and the flavors have combined.

7. Serve the eggplant and chickpea curry hot, topped with fresh cilantro.

Turkey Meatball and Spinach Pasta

This turkey meatball and spinach pasta is a protein-rich and nutritious dinner option that's ideal for refueling after a workout. With juicy turkey meatballs, tender spinach leaves, and al dente pasta tossed in a savory marinara sauce, this is a comforting and satisfying meal for the entire family to enjoy.

Serving Size: 4

Prep Time: 20 minutes

Cooking Time: 25 minutes

Ingredients:

- 1 pound ground turkey
- 1/2 cup breadcrumbs
- 1/4 cup grated Parmesan cheese
- 1 egg
- 2 cloves garlic, minced
- 1 teaspoon dried oregano
- 1 teaspoon dried basil
- Salt and pepper to taste
- 8 ounces pasta (such as spaghetti or penne)
- 2 cups fresh spinach leaves
- 2 cups marinara sauce
- Fresh basil for garnish

Instructions:

1. Preheat the oven to 375° Fahrenheit (190° Celsius).
2. In a large mixing bowl, combine the ground turkey, breadcrumbs, grated Parmesan cheese, egg, minced garlic, dried oregano, dried basil, salt, and pepper.
3. Mix until thoroughly combined.
4. Shape the turkey mixture into meatballs about an inch in diameter.
5. Place the meatballs on a baking sheet with parchment paper.
6. Bake meatballs in a preheated oven for 15-20 minutes, or until thoroughly cooked and lightly browned.
7. Meanwhile, cook the pasta according to the package instructions. Drain and set aside.
8. In a large skillet, heat the marinara sauce over medium heat.
9. Add the cooked meatballs and spinach leaves to the skillet.

10. Cook for about 5 minutes, or until the spinach has wilted and the meatballs are thoroughly heated.

11. Toss cooked pasta in the skillet until evenly coated with sauce.

12. Serve the turkey meatballs and spinach pasta hot, topped with fresh basil.

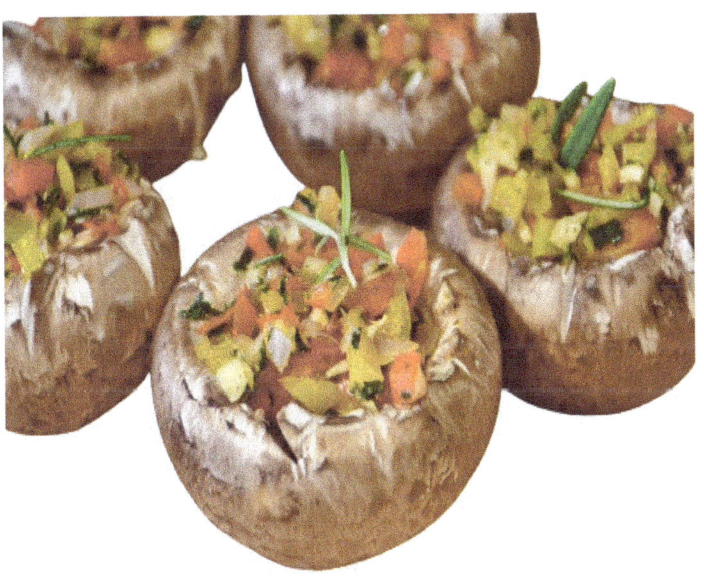

Chapter 5 : Power-Packed Snacks

Protein Energy Balls

These protein energy balls are ideal for a quick and nutritious snack on-the-go. They're high in protein, fiber, and healthy fats, and will keep you energized and satisfied in between meals.

Serving Size: Makes about 12 balls
Prep Time: 10 minutes

Ingredients:

- 1 cup rolled oats
- 1/2 cup almond butter
- 1/4 cup honey or maple syrup
- 1/4 cup chocolate chips
- 1/4 cup ground flaxseed
- 1 teaspoon vanilla extract

- Pinch of salt

Instructions:

1. In a mixing bowl, combine the rolled oats, almond butter, honey or maple syrup, chocolate chips, ground flaxseed, vanilla extract, and a pinch of salt.
2. Stir together all of the ingredients until they form a thick dough.
3. Roll the dough into tablespoon-sized balls and place on a lined baking sheet.
4. Refrigerate for at least 30 minutes to firm up.
5. Once chilled, place the energy balls in an airtight container for storage.
6. Enjoy one or two energy balls as a filling snack whenever you need a boost of energy!

Greek Yogurt Parfait

This Greek yogurt parfait is a delicious and nutritious snack high in protein and probiotics. It's a filling treat that's ideal for any time of day, thanks to the creamy Greek yogurt, fresh berries, and crunchy granola.

Serving Size: 1 parfait
Prep Time: 5 minutes

Ingredients:

1/2 cup Greek yogurt

1/4 cup fresh berries (such as strawberries, blueberries, or raspberries)

2 tablespoons granola

1 tablespoon honey (optional)

Instructions:

1. In a glass or bowl, place half of the Greek yogurt.
2. Place half of the fresh berries on top of the yogurt layer.
3. Sprinkle half of the granola over the berries.

4. Repeat layers with the remaining Greek yogurt, berries, and granola.

5. Drizzle with honey if desired for extra sweetness.

6. Enjoy your Greek yogurt parfait right away, or cover and refrigerate until ready to eat.

Avocado Toast with Egg

Avocado toast with egg is a nutritious and filling snack suitable for any time of day. Creamy avocado spread on whole grain toast, topped with a perfectly cooked egg, is a delicious and protein-rich treat.

Serving Size: 1 serving

Prep Time: 5 minutes

Cooking Time: 5 minutes

Ingredients:

- 1 slice whole grain bread, toasted
- 1/2 ripe avocado

- 1 large egg
- Salt and pepper to taste
- Optional toppings: sliced tomatoes, red pepper flakes, microgreens

Instructions:

1. In a small bowl, mash the ripe avocado with a fork until smooth.
2. Spread the mashed avocado evenly on the toasted whole grain bread.
3. Cook the egg in a nonstick skillet over medium heat until done to your liking.
4. Carefully transfer the cooked egg to the avocado toast.
5. Season with salt and pepper to taste.
6. Optional toppings include sliced tomatoes, red pepper flakes, and microgreens.
7. Enjoy avocado toast with egg as a tasty and nutritious snack!

Cottage Cheese and Fruit Bowl

This cottage cheese and fruit bowl is a protein-rich and refreshing snack that will help you feel full between meals. Creamy cottage cheese combined with sweet and juicy fruit makes for a tasty and nutritious snack.

Serving Size: 1 serving
Prep Time: 5 minutes

Ingredients:

- 1/2 cup cottage cheese
- 1/2 cup mixed fresh fruit (such as berries, pineapple, kiwi, or mango)
- 1 tablespoon honey or maple syrup (optional)
- 1 tablespoon chopped nuts or seeds (such as almonds, walnuts, or sunflower seeds)

Instructions:

1. Transfer the cottage cheese to a bowl.

2. Place the mixed fresh fruit on top of the cottage cheese.

3. Drizzle with honey or maple syrup if desired for extra sweetness.

4. Sprinkle with chopped nuts or seeds for added crunch and nutrition.

5. Enjoy your cottage cheese and fruit bowl as a quick and filling snack.

Turkey and Cheese Roll-Ups

These turkey and cheese roll-ups are a simple yet filling snack full of protein and flavor. Rolling slices of lean turkey breast around creamy cheese creates a tasty and nutritious snack that is ideal for on-the-go consumption.

Serving Size: Makes 4 roll-ups

Prep Time: 5 minutes

Ingredients:

- 4 slices deli turkey breast
- 4 slices cheese (such as cheddar, Swiss, or pepper jack)
- Mustard or mayonnaise (optional)
- Lettuce leaves (optional)
- Sliced tomatoes (optional)

Instructions:

1. Place a slice of deli turkey breast flat on a clean surface.
2. Place one slice of cheese on top of the turkey slice.
3. If desired, place a thin layer of mustard or mayonnaise on top of the cheese.
4. If desired, top with lettuce leaves and sliced tomatoes.
5. Roll the turkey slice tightly to contain the filling.

6. Secure with toothpicks if necessary to keep the roll-up together.

7. Repeat for the remaining turkey slices and filling ingredients.

Homemade Trail Mix

Homemade trail mix is a versatile and portable snack ideal for fueling your adventures. It's a delicious and nutritious treat that's simple to make and take with you wherever you go.

Serving Size: Makes about 2 cups
Prep Time: 5 minutes

Ingredients:
- 1/2 cup almonds
- 1/2 cup cashews
- 1/4 cup pumpkin seeds
- 1/4 cup dried cranberries
- 1/4 cup raisins

- 1/4 cup dark chocolate chips or chunks

Instructions:

1. In a mixing bowl, combine the almonds, cashews, pumpkin seeds, dried cranberries, raisins, and dark chocolate chips.
2. Stir until all the ingredients are well combined.
3. Transfer the trail mix to an airtight container or individual snack bags for easy transport.
4. Enjoy your homemade trail mix as a tasty and nutritious snack on-the-go!

Hummus and Veggie Sticks

Hummus and vegetable sticks are a classic and nutritious snack ideal for dipping and munching. Creamy hummus paired with crunchy fresh vegetables creates a delicious and satisfying treat that's packed with fiber, vitamins, and minerals..

Serving Size: 1 serving

Prep Time: 10 minutes

Ingredients:

- 1/2 cup hummus
- Assorted fresh vegetables for dipping (such as carrot sticks, cucumber slices, bell pepper strips, and cherry tomatoes)

Instructions:

1. Spoon the hummus into a small serving bowl.
2. Place the assorted fresh vegetables on a serving platter or plate.
3. Serve the hummus and vegetable sticks together for a tasty and nutritious snack!

Banana and Peanut Butter Sandwich

This banana and peanut butter sandwich is a simple and filling snack for any time of day. Creamy peanut butter spread on whole grain bread, topped with sliced banana, is a tasty and nutritious snack high in protein, fiber, and good fats.

Serving Size: 1 sandwich

Prep Time: 5 minutes

Ingredients:

- 2 slices whole grain bread
- 2 tablespoons peanut butter
- 1 ripe banana, sliced

Instructions:

1. Spread peanut butter evenly over a slice of whole grain bread.
2. Place sliced bananas on top of the peanut butter.
3. Place the second slice of whole grain bread on top to make a sandwich.
4. If desired, cut the sandwich in half and eat as a quick and satisfying snack!

Edamame with Sea Salt

Edamame with sea salt is a nutritious and flavorful snack ideal for on-the-go consumption. Steamed edamame pods sprinkled with sea salt are a delicious and protein-packed snack that is both satisfying and simple to prepare.

Serving Size: 1 serving
Prep Time: 5 minutes
Cooking Time: 5 minutes

Ingredients:

- 1 cup frozen edamame pods
- Sea salt, to taste

Instructions:

1. Bring a pot of water to a boil on high heat.

2. Add the frozen edamame pods to the boiling water and cook for 3-5 minutes, or until tender.

3. Drain the cooked edamame pods and place them in a serving bowl.

4. Toss in sea salt to taste, and coat well.

5. Serve edamame with sea salt hot or at room temperature for a tasty and nutritious snack!

Chia Seed Pudding

Chia seed pudding is a creamy, nutritious snack that will satisfy your sweet tooth. Made with chia seeds, almond milk, and a touch of sweetness, it's a tasty and versatile treat that you can customize with your favorite toppings.

Serving Size: Makes 2 servings

Prep Time: 5 minutes

Ingredients:

- 1/4 cup chia seeds
- 1 cup almond milk (or any milk of your choice)
- 1 tablespoon honey or maple syrup (optional)
- 1/2 teaspoon vanilla extract
- Fresh fruit, nuts, seeds, or granola for topping (optional)

Instructions:

1. In a mixing bowl or jar, combine the chia seeds, almond milk, honey or maple syrup (if using), and vanilla extract.
2. Stir until all the ingredients are well combined.
3. Cover the bowl or jar and chill for at least 2 hours, or overnight, to allow the chia seeds to absorb the liquid and thicken into pudding.
4. Once chilled and set, stir the chia seed pudding to dislodge any lumps.

5. Serve the chia seed pudding in individual bowls or jars, garnished with your favorite fresh fruit, nuts, seeds, or granola if desired.

6. Enjoy your chia seed pudding as a tasty and nutritious snack.

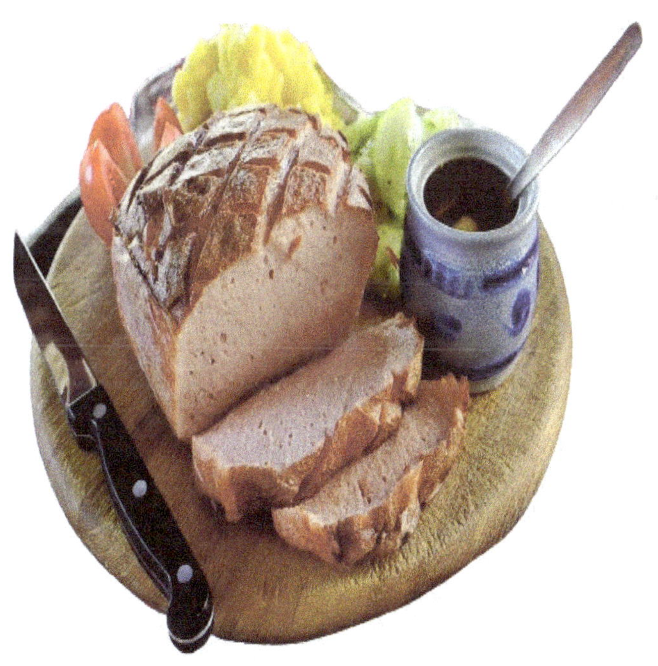

Chapter 6 : EnergizingSnacks for Between Meals

Apple and Peanut Butter Slices

Apple and peanut butter slices are a traditional and energizing snack that is ideal for refueling between meals. Crisp apple slices combined with creamy peanut butter make a delicious and satisfying treat high in fiber, protein, and healthy fats.

Serving Size: 1 serving
Prep Time: 5 minutes

Ingredients:

- 1 apple, cored and sliced
- 2 tablespoons peanut butter

Instructions:

1. Core the apple and cut it into thin wedges.

2. Spread peanut butter over one side of each apple slice.

3. Stack the apple slices to create mini sandwiches.

4. Enjoy apple and peanut butter slices as a quick and energizing snack!

Greek Yogurt and Berries Bowl

Greek yogurt and berry bowl is a refreshing and nutritious snack that will satisfy your hunger between meals. Creamy Greek yogurt combined with sweet and juicy berries creates a tasty and energizing treat high in protein, vitamins, and antioxidants.

Serving Size: 1 serving

Prep Time: 5 minutes

Ingredients:

1. 1/2 cup Greek yogurt

2. 1/2 cup mixed berries (such as strawberries, blueberries, and raspberries)

3. 1 tablespoon honey or maple syrup (optional)

4. 1 tablespoon sliced almonds or chopped walnuts (optional)

Instructions:

1. Spoon Greek yogurt into a serving bowl.

2. Garnish with mixed berries.

3. Drizzle with honey or maple syrup if desired for extra sweetness.

4. Sprinkle with sliced almonds or chopped walnuts for added crunch and nutrition.

5. Enjoy your Greek yogurt and berry bowl for a quick and energizing snack!

Trail Mix Energy Bars

Trail mix energy bars are a homemade and nutritious snack that is ideal for fueling your adventures.

They're a delicious and energizing treat that's simple to make and take with you wherever you go.

Serving Size: Makes 8 bars
Prep Time: 10 minutes
Cooking Time: 20 minutes

Ingredients:

- 1 cup rolled oats
- 1/2 cup mixed nuts and seeds (such as almonds, cashews, pumpkin seeds, and sunflower seeds)
- 1/2 cup dried fruit (such as raisins, cranberries, or chopped apricots)
- 1/4 cup honey or maple syrup
- 1/4 cup almond butter or peanut butter
- 1/4 cup chocolate chips or chunks (optional)

Instructions:

1. Preheat the oven to 350°F (175°C). Line an 8x8-inch baking pan with parchment paper, leaving an overhang on each side for easy removal.

2. In a large mixing bowl, combine the rolled oats, mixed nuts and seeds, dried fruit, and chocolate chips (if desired).

3. In a small saucepan, combine honey or maple syrup and almond butter or peanut butter over low heat, stirring until melted and smooth.

4. Pour the melted mixture into the mixing bowl and combine with the dry ingredients.

5. Stir until the ingredients are well combined and evenly coated.

6. Transfer the mixture to the prepared baking pan and press firmly to compact.

7. Bake in the preheated oven for 20-25 minutes, or until golden brown and set.

8. Remove from the oven and allow to cool completely in the pan.

9. Once cooled, remove the bars from the pan using the parchment paper overhang and cut into 8 bars.

10. Keep trail mix energy bars in an airtight container at room temperature for up to a week.

11. Enjoy this homemade and energizing snack on the go!

Banana and Almond Butter Rice Cakes

Banana and Almond Butter Rice cakes are a quick and satisfying snack that is ideal for busy days. Crispy rice cakes topped with creamy almond butter and sliced banana are a delicious and energizing treat full of fiber, protein, and healthy fats.

Serving Size: 1 serving

Prep Time: 5 minutes

Ingredients:

- 1 rice cake

- 1 tablespoon almond butter

- 1/2 banana, sliced

Instructions:

1. Spread almond butter evenly across the top of the rice cake.

2. Place sliced bananas on top of the almond butter.

3. Enjoy your banana and almond butter rice cake for a quick and energizing snack!

Homemade Granola Bars

Homemade granola bars are a nutritious and filling snack that is ideal for fueling your busy days. They're a delicious and energizing treat that you can customize with your favorite ingredients.

Serving Size: Makes 12 bars
Prep Time: 10 minutes

Cooking Time: 20 minutes

Ingredients:

- 2 cups rolled oats
- 1/2 cup mixed nuts and seeds (such as almonds, walnuts, pumpkin seeds, and sunflower seeds)
- 1/2 cup dried fruit (such as raisins, cranberries, or chopped apricots)
- 1/4 cup honey or maple syrup
- 1/4 cup almond butter or peanut butter
- 1/4 cup coconut oil, melted
- 1 teaspoon vanilla extract
- Pinch of salt

Instructions:

1. Preheat the oven to 350°F (175°C). Line an 8x8-inch baking pan with parchment paper, leaving an overhang on each side for easy removal.

2. In a large mixing bowl, combine the rolled oats, nuts, seeds, and dried fruit.

3. In a small saucepan, combine honey or maple syrup, almond butter or peanut butter, coconut oil, vanilla extract, and a pinch of salt over low heat. Stir until melted and smooth.

4. Pour the melted mixture into the mixing bowl and combine with the dry ingredients.

5. Stir until the ingredients are well combined and evenly coated.

6. Transfer the mixture to the prepared baking pan and press firmly to compact.

7. Bake in the preheated oven for 20-25 minutes, or until golden brown and set.

8. Remove from the oven and allow to cool completely in the pan.

9. Once cooled, remove the bars from the pan using the parchment paper overhang and cut into 12 bars.

10. Once cooled, remove the bars from the pan using the parchment paper overhang and cut into 12 bars.

11. Keep homemade granola bars in an airtight container at room temperature for up to a week.

12. Enjoy this homemade and energizing snack on the go!

Cucumber and Hummus Slices

Cucumber and hummus slices are a refreshing and nutritious snack that will satisfy your hunger in between meals. Crisp cucumber slices combined with creamy hummus make a tasty and energizing snack high in fiber, protein, and vitamins.

Serving Size: 1 serving
Prep Time: 5 minutes

Ingredients:

1/2 cucumber, sliced

2 tablespoons hummus

Instructions:

1. Slice the cucumber into thin rounds.

2. Spread hummus onto one side of each cucumber slice.

3. Enjoy cucumber and hummus slices as a quick and energizing snack!

Chocolate Avocado Smoothie

Chocolate avocado smoothie is a creamy and decadent snack that will satisfy your sweet cravings. It's a tasty and energizing treat full of nutrients and flavor, made with ripe avocado, cocoa powder, banana, and almond milk.

Serving Size: 1 serving

Prep Time: 5 minutes

Ingredients:

- 1/2 ripe avocado

- 1 tablespoon cocoa powder

- 1/2 ripe banana

- 1 cup almond milk

- 1 tablespoon honey or maple syrup (optional)

- Ice cubes (optional)

Instructions:

- Put the flesh of a ripe avocado into a blender.

- Combine the cocoa powder, ripe banana, almond milk, and honey or maple syrup (if using).

- Blend until smooth and creamy.

- If desired, add ice cubes to create a chilled and refreshing smoothie.

- Pour into a glass and enjoy your chocolate avocado smoothie as a tasty and energizing snack.

Quinoa Salad Cups

Quinoa salad cups are a portable and nutritious snack that is ideal for taking on the go. Quinoa cooked with vegetables and herbs served in lettuce cups is a delicious and energizing treat high in protein, fiber, and vitamins.

Serving Size: Makes 4 cups
Prep Time: 15 minutes
Cooking Time: 15 minutes

Ingredients:

- 1 cup cooked quinoa
- 1/2 cup cherry tomatoes, diced
- 1/2 cucumber, diced
- 1/4 cup red onion, finely chopped
- 1/4 cup fresh parsley, chopped
- Juice of 1 lemon
- 2 tablespoons olive oil

- Salt and pepper to taste

- 4 large lettuce leaves (such as romaine or butter lettuce)

Instructions:

1. In a mixing bowl, combine cooked quinoa, cherry tomatoes, cucumber, red onion, and fresh parsley.

2. Drizzle with lemon juice and olive oil.

3. Season with salt and pepper to taste.

4. Stir until all the ingredients are well combined.

5. Spoon the quinoa salad mixture into lettuce leaves to make cups.

6. Serve the quinoa salad cups immediately, or cover and chill until ready to eat.

7. Enjoy as a portable, energizing snack!

Tuna Salad Stuffed Bell Peppers

Tuna salad stuffed bell peppers are a protein-rich and filling snack that is ideal for refueling in between meals. Creamy tuna salad stuffed into crisp bell pepper halves is a delicious and energizing treat that's simple to prepare and enjoy.

Serving Size: Makes 4 halves
Prep Time: 10 minutes

Ingredients:

- 1 can tuna, drained
- 1/4 cup Greek yogurt or mayonnaise
- 1 tablespoon Dijon mustard
- 1/4 cup diced celery
- 1/4 cup diced red onion
- Salt and pepper to taste
- 2 bell peppers, halved and seeded

Instructions:

1. In a mixing bowl, combine the drained tuna, Greek yogurt or mayonnaise, Dijon mustard, diced celery, and red onion.

2. Season with salt and pepper to taste.

3. Stir until the ingredients are well combined and evenly coated.

4. Spoon the tuna salad into bell pepper halves.

5. Serve the tuna salad stuffed bell peppers immediately, or cover and chill until ready to eat.

6. Enjoy as a protein-rich, energizing snack!

Sweet Potato Toast with Avocado

Sweet potato toast with avocado is a healthy and filling snack for any time of day. Roasted sweet potato slices topped with creamy avocado and sea salt are a tasty and energizing snack high in fiber, vitamins, and healthy fats.

Serving Size: 1 serving

Prep Time: 10 minutes

Cooking Time: 15 minutes

Ingredients:

- 1 medium sweet potato, sliced into 1/4 inch thick rounds
- 1 ripe avocado, sliced
- Sea salt to taste
- Optional toppings: red pepper flakes, microgreens, sliced radishes

Instructions:

1. Preheat the oven to 400° F (200° C). Line a baking sheet with parchment paper.
2. Place sweet potato slices in a single layer on the prepared baking sheet.
3. Bake in the preheated oven for 15-20 minutes, flipping halfway through, or until

sweet potato slices are tender and lightly browned.

4. Remove from the oven and allow to cool slightly.

5. Top each sweet potato slice with sliced avocado.

6. Season with sea salt to taste.

7. Optional toppings include red pepper flakes, microgreens, and sliced radishes.

8. Enjoy your sweet potato toast with avocado as a tasty and energizing snack!

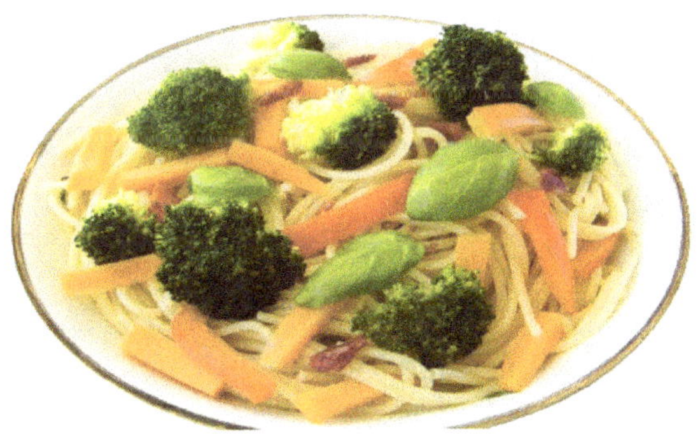

Chapter 7: Protein-Rich Smoothies and Shakes

Berry Blast Protein Smoothie

This Berry Blast Protein Smoothie is a tasty and nutritious way to begin the day or refuel after a workout. It's a refreshing treat full of antioxidants from mixed berries and protein from Greek yogurt, keeping you satisfied and energized.

Serving Size: 1 smoothie
Prep Time: 5 minutes

Ingredients:

- 1/2 cup mixed berries (strawberries, blueberries, raspberries)
- 1/2 cup Greek yogurt
- 1/2 cup almond milk
- 1 scoop vanilla protein powder

- 1 tablespoon honey (optional)
- Ice cubes (optional)

Instructions:

1. Mix the berries, Greek yogurt, almond milk, protein powder, and honey (if using) in a blender.
2. Blend until smooth and creamy.
3. If you prefer a colder consistency, add some ice cubes.
4. Pour into a glass and enjoy the Berry Blast Protein Smoothie!

Banana Peanut Butter Protein Shake

This Banana Peanut Butter Protein Shake is a classic flavor combination that makes for a quick and satisfying snack. With a creamy banana texture and a rich peanut butter flavor, this protein-packed treat will keep you satisfied for hours.

Serving Size: 1 shake

Prep Time: 5 minutes

Ingredients:

- 1 ripe banana
- 2 tablespoons peanut butter
- 1 cup milk (dairy or plant-based)
- 1 scoop chocolate protein powder
- Ice cubes (optional)

Instructions:

1. Peel the banana and put it in a blender.
2. Pour the peanut butter, milk, protein powder, and ice cubes (if using) into the blender.
3. Blend until smooth and creamy.
4. Pour into a glass and enjoy the Banana Peanut Butter Protein Shake!

Green Goddess Protein Smoothie

The Green Goddess Protein Smoothie is a refreshing and nutritious way to incorporate more greens into your diet. It's a creamy and delicious smoothie that contains spinach, banana, and protein-rich Greek yogurt, leaving you feeling energized and satisfied.

Serving Size: 1 smoothie

Prep Time: 5 minutes

Ingredients:

- 1 cup fresh spinach leaves
- 1/2 ripe banana
- 1/2 cup Greek yogurt
- 1/2 cup almond milk
- 1 scoop vanilla protein powder
- 1 tablespoon honey (optional)
- Ice cubes (optional)

Instructions:

1. Combine spinach leaves, banana, Greek yogurt, almond milk, protein powder, and honey (if using) in a blender.
2. Blend until smooth and creamy.
3. If you prefer a colder consistency, add some ice cubes.
4. Pour into a glass and enjoy the Green Goddess Protein Smoothie!

Chocolate Almond Protein Shake

Satisfy your chocolate cravings with this Chocolate Almond Protein Shake. With the rich flavor of cocoa powder and the nutty flavor of almonds, this protein-packed shake is a delicious and satisfying treat for any time of day.

Serving Size: 1 shake
Prep Time: 5 minutes

Ingredients:

- 1 cup almond milk
- 1 scoop chocolate protein powder
- 1 tablespoon almond butter
- 1 teaspoon cocoa powder
- 1/2 teaspoon vanilla extract
- Ice cubes (optional)

Instructions:

1. In a blender, combine almond milk, chocolate protein powder, almond butter, cocoa powder, vanilla extract, and ice cubes (optional).
2. Blend until smooth and creamy.
3. Pour into a glass and enjoy the chocolate.

Tropical Paradise Protein Smoothie

Travel to the tropics with this Tropical Paradise Protein Smoothie. This protein-rich smoothie, which includes pineapple, mango, and coconut, is like a vacation in a glass. Ideal for breakfast or a post-workout refuel!

Serving Size: 1 smoothie

Prep Time: 5 minutes

Ingredients:

- 1/2 cup frozen pineapple chunks
- 1/2 cup frozen mango chunks
- 1/2 cup coconut milk
- 1/2 cup Greek yogurt
- 1 scoop vanilla protein powder
- 1 tablespoon shredded coconut (optional)
- Ice cubes (optional)

Instructions:

1. In a blender, combine frozen pineapple chunks, frozen mango chunks, coconut milk, Greek yogurt, protein powder, shredded coconut (optional), and ice cubes.

2. Blend until smooth and creamy.

3. Pour in a glass and enjoy your Tropical Paradise Protein Smoothie!

Blueberry Banana Protein Smoothie Bowl

This Blueberry Banana Protein Smoothie Bowl is a delicious and satisfying way to begin the day. Topped with crunchy granola and fresh fruit, this protein-packed breakfast will keep you energized and fueled for hours.

Serving Size: 1 smoothie bowl
Prep Time: 5 minutes

Ingredients:

- 1/2 cup frozen blueberries
- 1/2 ripe banana
- 1/2 cup almond milk

- 1/2 cup Greek yogurt
- 1 scoop vanilla protein powder
- Toppings: granola, fresh blueberries, sliced banana, chia seeds

Instructions:

1. Combine frozen blueberries, banana, almond milk, Greek yogurt, and protein powder in a blender.
2. Blend until smooth and creamy.
3. Pour the smoothie into a bowl.
4. Garnish with granola, fresh blueberries, sliced banana, and chia seeds.
5. Enjoy your Blueberry Banana Protein Smoothie Bowl with a spoon.

Peanut Butter Banana Protein Shake

The classic Peanut Butter Banana Protein Shake never disappoints. With a creamy banana texture and the nutty flavor of peanut butter, this protein-rich shake will keep you satisfied and fueled for hours.

Serving Size: 1 shake

Prep Time: 5 minutes

Ingredients:

- 1 ripe banana
- 2 tablespoons peanut butter
- 1 cup milk (dairy or plant-based)
- 1 scoop vanilla protein powder
- Ice cubes (optional)

Instructions:

1. Peel the banana and put it in a blender.
2. Pour the peanut butter, milk, protein powder, and ice cubes (if using) into the blender.
3. Blend until smooth and creamy.
4. Pour in a glass and enjoy your Peanut Butter Banana Protein Shake!

Mocha Protein Frappuccino

Enjoy the rich flavor of coffee with this Mocha Protein Frappuccino. Made with cold brew coffee, cocoa powder, and protein powder, this refreshing and energizing drink is ideal for a midday pick-me-up.

Serving Size: 1 frappuccino
Prep Time: 5 minutes

Ingredients:

- 1 cup cold brew coffee
- 1/2 cup milk (dairy or plant-based)
- 1 scoop chocolate protein powder
- 1 tablespoon cocoa powder
- 1 tablespoon honey or maple syrup (optional)
- Ice cubes

Instructions:

1. In a blender, combine cold brew coffee, milk, chocolate protein powder, cocoa powder, honey or maple syrup (if desired), and ice cubes.

2. Blend until smooth and creamy.

3. Pour in a glass and enjoy your Mocha Protein Frappuccino!

Vanilla Almond Protein Shake

The Vanilla Almond Protein Shake is a simple but tasty way to refuel after a workout. With the sweet flavor of vanilla and the nutty flavor of almonds, this protein-packed shake will keep you satisfied and fueled for hours.

Serving Size: 1 shake

Prep Time: 5 minutes

Ingredients:

- 1 cup almond milk

- 1 scoop vanilla protein powder
- 1/4 teaspoon almond extract
- 1 tablespoon almond butter
- Ice cubes (optional)

Instructions:

1. In a blender, combine almond milk, vanilla protein powder, almond extract, almond butter, and ice cubes (if desired).
2. Blend until smooth and creamy.
3. Pour in a glass and enjoy your Vanilla Almond Protein Shake!

Chocolate Cherry Protein Smoothie

Enjoy the sweet and tart flavors of chocolate and cherry with this Chocolate Cherry Protein Smoothie. It's a delicious and satisfying treat that's high in antioxidants and protein, making it ideal for any time of the day.

Serving Size: 1 smoothie

Prep Time: 5 minutes

Ingredients:

- 1/2 cup frozen cherries
- 1 tablespoon cocoa powder
- 1/2 cup Greek yogurt
- 1/2 cup almond milk
- 1 scoop chocolate protein powder
- 1 tablespoon honey (optional)
- Ice cubes (optional)

Instructions:

1. Combine frozen cherries, cocoa powder, Greek yogurt, almond milk, protein powder, and honey (if using) in a blender.
2. Blend until smooth and creamy.
3. If you prefer a colder consistency, add some ice cubes.

4. Pour in a glass and enjoy your Chocolate Cherry Protein Smoothie!

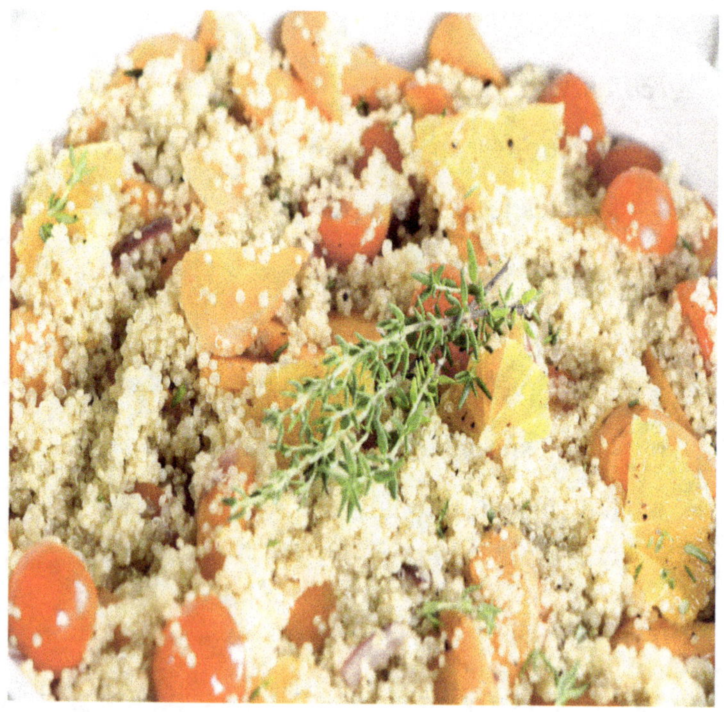

Chapter 8: Meal Planning and Prep

Effective Meal Planning Strategies

Meal planning is more than just deciding what to eat each week; it is a strategic approach to nourishing your body efficiently and effectively. Here are some key strategies to consider as you embark on your meal planning journey:

Set Clear Goals: Before you begin meal planning, make sure your goals are clear and attainable. Whether you want to gain muscle, improve endurance, or simply maintain good health, your meal plan should reflect these goals.

Balance Macronutrients: A well-balanced meal plan includes carbohydrates, proteins, and fats that are tailored to your specific needs and goals. Include lean proteins, complex carbohydrates, and healthy fats in each meal to promote muscle growth, energy production, and overall health.

Prioritize Nutrient-Dense Foods: Fill your plate with fruits, vegetables, whole grains, and lean proteins. These foods not only provide essential vitamins and minerals, but also help with satiety and overall well-being.

Plan ahead: Set aside time each week to plan your meals and snacks. Whether you prefer to use a meal planning app, spreadsheet, or the old-fashioned pen and paper, having a plan in place can help you stay on track and avoid impulsive food purchases.

Preparing Ingredients in Advance: To make meal preparation easier during busy weekdays, consider prepping ingredients ahead of time. Cut vegetables, cook grains, and portion out snacks on weekends or during downtime to save time and effort during the week.

Maintain Flexibility: While having a meal plan in place is beneficial, it is critical to remain flexible and adaptable. Life is unpredictable, and you may need to adjust your meals or swap ingredients due to availability or changing circumstances.

By implementing these meal planning strategies, you can gain control of your nutrition and position yourself for success both inside and outside of the gym.

Batch Cooking for Athletes

For athletes and fitness enthusiasts, batch cooking can be a game changer when it comes to meal planning. Batch cooking is the process of preparing large amounts of food ahead of time and portioning it out for multiple meals throughout the week. Here's why batch cooking is especially beneficial to athletes:

Time Efficiency: Athletes frequently have demanding training schedules that leave little time for meal prep. Batch cooking enables you to save time by preparing multiple meals at once, reducing the need for daily cooking sessions.

Consistency is essential for proper nutrition and performance. Batch cooking your meals ensures that your body receives the nutrients it requires to function properly.

Portion Control: Batch cooking allows you to portion out your meals ahead of time, which helps you stay on track and avoid overeating. This is especially useful for athletes who need to closely monitor their calorie intake and macronutrient ratios.

Variety and Convenience: Batch cooking does not require eating the same meal every day. With careful planning, you can prepare a variety of dishes while incorporating different flavors and ingredients into them. Simply store them in the refrigerator or freezer, and you'll have convenient and nutritious options on hand whenever hunger strikes.

Cost Savings: Cooking in bulk can result in long-term cost savings. You can reduce food waste and lower your overall grocery bill by buying in bulk and using ingredients efficiently.

Incorporating batch cooking into your meal prep routine can help streamline your nutrition efforts, allowing you to devote more time and energy to your training and performance objectives.

Chapter 9: Eating for Your Goals

Eating for Your Goals isn't a one-size-fits-all approach; it's about tailoring your nutrition to your specific goals, whether they're building muscle, optimizing fat loss, or improving overall wellness. In this chapter, we'll look at how to tailor your diet to your specific goals, with a focus on strategies for muscle gain and fat loss.

Customizing Nutrition for Muscle Gain

Muscle gain necessitates a combination of good nutrition, resistance training, and enough rest. Here are some important strategies for customizing your nutrition to promote muscle growth:

Caloric Surplus: To gain muscle, you must consume more calories than you expend, resulting in a caloric surplus. Consume nutrient-dense foods with a balanced macronutrient profile (proteins, carbohydrates, and fats) to fuel your workouts and promote muscle repair and growth.

Protein is the foundation of muscle, so it's critical to prioritize high-quality protein sources like lean meats, poultry, fish, eggs, dairy, legumes, and plant-based protein sources like tofu and tempeh. To support muscle protein synthesis, include protein in all meals and snacks.

Carbohydrate Fuel: Carbohydrates provide energy for strenuous exercise and replenish glycogen stores in muscles. Include complex carbohydrates in your diet, such as whole grains, fruits, vegetables, and legumes, to fuel your workouts and promote recovery.

Healthy Fats: While protein and carbohydrates are necessary for muscle growth, don't underestimate the role of healthy fats. Avocados, nuts, seeds, olive oil, and fatty fish are all good sources of healthy fats that help with hormone production, joint health, and overall well-being.

Timing and Distribution: Spread out your meals and snacks evenly throughout the day to ensure a consistent supply of nutrients to your muscles. To maximize muscle repair and recovery, consume a combination of protein and carbohydrates before and after your workouts.

By implementing these strategies and prioritizing nutrient-dense foods, you can create an ideal environment for muscle growth and development.

Optimizing Nutrition for Fat Loss

Fat loss necessitates a strategic approach to nutrition that emphasizes creating a calorie deficit while maintaining muscle mass. Here are some important strategies for optimizing your diet for fat loss:

Caloric Deficit: To lose fat, you must eat fewer calories than you expend, resulting in a caloric deficit. To avoid muscle loss and nutrient deficiencies, it is necessary to do so gradually and consistently.

Protein Priority: Protein aids in fat loss by maintaining lean muscle mass and promoting feelings of fullness. Include lean protein sources in every meal and snack to promote satiety, muscle retention, and metabolic rate.

Balanced Macronutrients: While cutting calories, don't ignore carbohydrates and fats completely. Instead, concentrate on consuming a variety of macronutrients to maintain energy levels, hormonal balance, and overall well-being. To fuel your body efficiently, consume complex carbohydrates, healthy fats, and lean proteins.

Portion Control: Pay attention to portion sizes and eat mindfully to avoid overeating. Use measuring cups, food scales, and portion control plates to accurately manage portion sizes and track your calorie intake.

Whole Foods Emphasis: Choose whole, minimally processed foods over highly processed and refined alternatives. Whole foods are more nutrient dense, satisfying, and promote fat loss than processed foods. Fill your plate with fruits, vegetables, lean proteins, whole grains, and healthy fats to help you lose weight.

Hydration and Fiber: Stay hydrated and eat plenty of fiber-rich foods to improve digestion, satiety, and overall health. Drink plenty of water throughout the day and eat fiber-rich foods like fruits, vegetables, whole grains, legumes, and nuts to keep you full and satisfied.

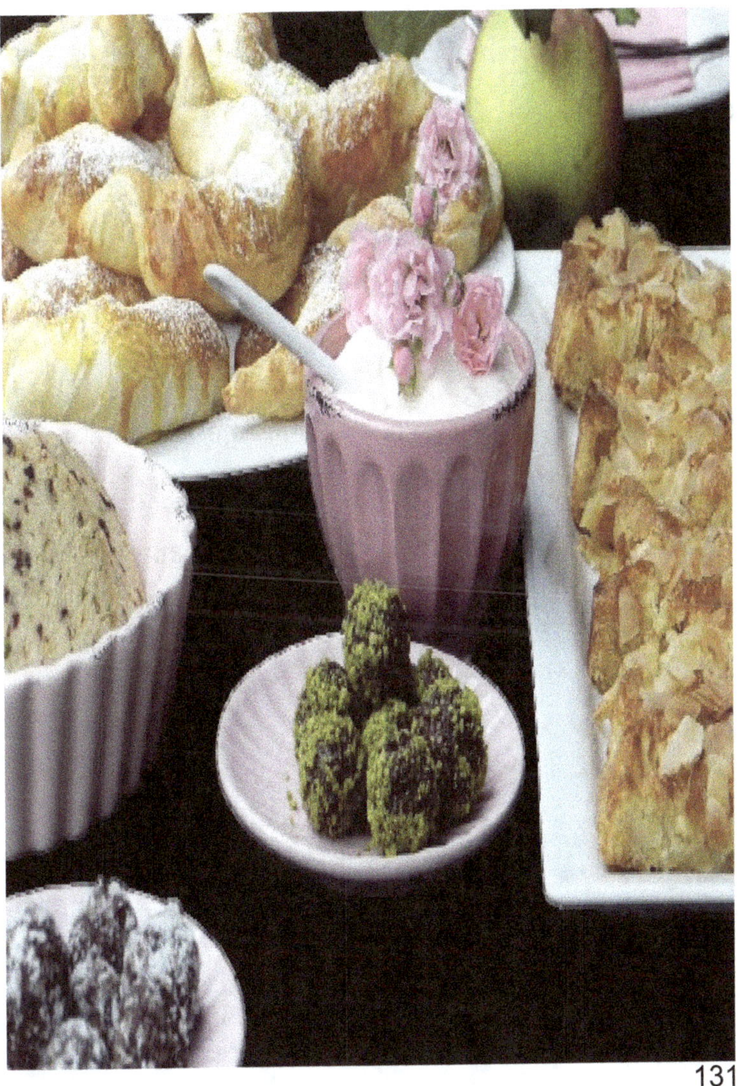

Chapter 10 : Staying on Track

Staying on track is often the most difficult aspect of achieving our health and fitness goals. Chapter 10 focuses on practical strategies for overcoming common obstacles, such as dining out and social events, while remaining balanced and sustainable in our approach to nutrition and lifestyle.

Tips for Dining and Social Events

Eating out or attending social gatherings can make it difficult to stick to our nutrition goals. However, with the right strategies in place, we can enjoy these experiences while remaining committed to our health goals. Here are some tips for eating out and attending social events:

Plan Ahead: Before going to a restaurant or event, review the menu or ask about the food options. Look for dishes that fit your dietary preferences and goals, such as grilled proteins, salads, and vegetable-based options.

Make Substitutions: Do not be afraid to request changes to your meal to make it healthier. Request steamed vegetables instead of fries, grilled or baked proteins instead of fried, and dressings and sauces on the side to keep portions under control.

Practice Portion Control: Restaurant portions are typically larger than those we might consume at home. Consider sharing a meal with a friend or family member, or request a take-out box to portion out half of your meal before you begin eating.

Be Mindful of Beverages: Be mindful of your beverage choices, as they can add a significant number of calories and sugar to your meal. Rather than sugary sodas or alcoholic beverages, choose water, unsweetened tea, or other low-calorie options.

Focus on Socializing: While food is frequently an important part of social gatherings, try to shift the emphasis away from eating and toward enjoying the company of friends and loved ones. Engage in conversation, participate in activities, and consider the overall experience rather than just the food.

Allow yourself to eat your favorite foods in moderation, without feeling guilty or deprived. It's okay to indulge on occasion, as long as it's balanced with healthy eating habits and regular exercise.

Maintaining Balance and Sustainability

Maintaining balance and sustainability is critical for long-term success in any nutrition and fitness journey. Here are some approaches to achieving balance and sustainability:

Flexible Eating: Take a flexible approach to eating that allows you to enjoy a variety of foods while still meeting your nutritional requirements. Instead of strict dieting or rigid meal plans, concentrate on eating nutritious foods most of the time while allowing for occasional treats.

Listen to Your Body: Recognize your body's hunger and fullness cues and eat intuitively. Eat when you're hungry and stop when you're full, rather than following strict meal times or portion sizes dictated by outside influences.

Find Joy in Movement: Rather than viewing exercise as a chore, seek out physical activities that you enjoy and that bring you pleasure. Make movement a fun and integral part of your lifestyle by dancing, hiking, practicing yoga, or participating in sports.

Be Kind to Yourself: Throughout your journey, practice self-compassion. Accept that setbacks and challenges are normal parts of the process, and concentrate on progress rather than perfection.

Celebrate Non-Scale Victories: Instead of focusing on the number on the scale, celebrate other indicators of success such as increased energy, improved mood, strength gains, and overall health.

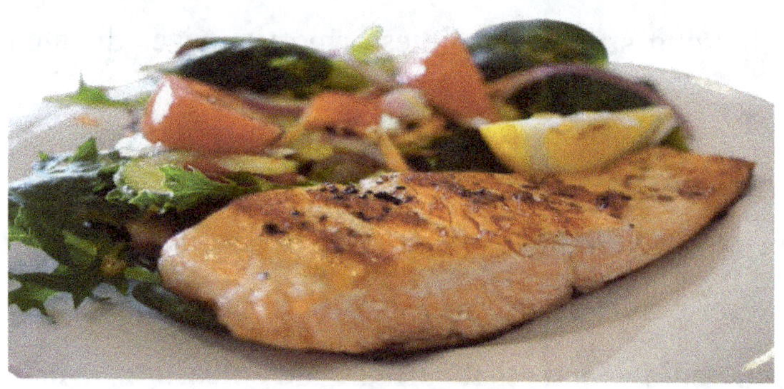

Conclusion

Additional Resources

In addition to the wealth of information and guidance provided in the Bodybuilding Diet Cookbook for Women, there are several other resources available to supplement and enhance the reader's journey to optimal health and fitness. These resources build on the principles outlined in the cookbook, offering additional education, support, and inspiration to women looking to transform their bodies and lives through nutrition and exercise.

Online Communities and Forums: Women embarking on their bodybuilding journey can benefit from online fitness and nutrition communities and forums. These communities allow women to connect with like-minded people, share their experiences, ask questions, and seek advice from experts and other enthusiasts. Whether it's a Facebook group, subreddit, or dedicated forum, these online communities provide a safe and encouraging space for women to learn and grow on their fitness journey.

Nutrition and Fitness Apps: In today's digital age, there are numerous nutrition and fitness apps available to help women track their progress, plan their meals, and stay accountable to their goals. These apps, which include calorie counting, workout trackers, and meal planning tools, provide women with a convenient and accessible way to stay on track with their bodybuilding diet and fitness regimen. Popular apps include MyFitnessPal, Fitbit, and Lifesum, among others.

Nutrition and fitness coaching can be a valuable resource for women looking for personalised guidance and support on their bodybuilding journey.

Working with a qualified coach or personal trainer can provide women with personalized guidance, accountability, and motivation to help them achieve their goals more effectively. There are a variety of options to suit different preferences and budgets, including one-on-one coaching sessions, online coaching programs, and group coaching programs.

Books & Educational Resources: In addition to the Bodybuilding Diet Cookbook for Women, there are numerous books and educational resources available to help women improve their knowledge of nutrition, fitness, and bodybuilding. These resources cover macronutrient manipulation, meal planning, supplementation, and other topics, giving you a thorough understanding of the principles and practices of bodybuilding nutrition. Some recommended books are "The New Rules of Lifting for Women" by Lou Schuler and Alwyn Cosgrove, "Strong Curves" by Bret Contreras and Kellie Davis, and "Bigger Leaner Stronger" by Michael Matthews, among others.

Online Courses and Workshops: For women who prefer a more structured and comprehensive learning experience, online courses and workshops allow them to delve deeper into the world of bodybuilding nutrition and fitness. These courses are usually led by experienced coaches and experts in the field, and they cover topics like meal planning, macronutrient tracking, workout programming, and more. Whether it's a short-term workshop or a longer certification program, these courses offer valuable education and practical skills to help women on their bodybuilding journey.